My Metabolic Miracle
by Cyndi Overton
Smashwords Edition
Copyright 2014 Overton Publishing

Smashwords Edition, License Notes

Acknowledgment

I thank God for his unconditional love.

I thank my handsome and adoring husband for loving me, for pushing me to write this book and for supporting me in every way, every day of our lives.

I thank my children for their love and support. I could not have been blessed with better!

Lastly, I thank Diane Kress, author of Metabolism Miracle. Through her book, she has given me a chance to help myself and others. For that, I am forever grateful.

Foreword

My family is deeply spiritual. Through prayer and listening to our "voices" deep within we are guided every day by our connection with God. Our absolute faith has carried us through very difficult times in our lives, given us answers when there seemingly were none and has literally saved our lives. This is the story of how absolute faith saved my life, saved my husbands life, saved my role as a mom and a wife and helped me make the world a better place by helping others.

I will never forget the day I sat to scroll through a favorite Facebook site of mine, Thyroid Sexy. A post written by a woman desperately asking for help displayed on the screen. As I read the symptoms she described I remember thinking she could be me. I, too, was desperate so I clicked to read the comments. In retrospect, I wish I had taken a screen shot of that post and the comment that forever changed my life. Two simple words shown on the screen METABOLISM MIRACLE. Looking back, it's as if there was a golden glow around those words. This was the first time I saw them together. I used both of them daily. As my husband and I struggled with metabolism issues, we were extremely blessed with miracles, as well. However, these two words together was something special! Something distracted me and I never got back to that post. Those two words kept popping into my head. Later that evening I did an internet search. I typed the words into my search engine and was brought to another world, a world of hope! I vividly remember thanking God for showing me the post and for keeping the words ALIVE in my head.

Metabolism Miracle is a book written by Diane Kress. Her book explains her plan and her story of how she developed the plan. My book, My Metabolic Miracle is my story. Being completely honest and transparent from behind this computer screen is very important to me and very difficult considering the subject. I am disclosing information that most women lie about their whole lives. However, helping more people supersedes my ego. I look forward to opening a dialogue with readers to raise awareness about this debilitating illness known as Metabolism B.

The Beginning

A year ago this book began as a blog, Simply Cynful. You see, I wanted to write. I had many things I wanted to write about but needed to find something I "needed" to write about. My thought was to assign a topic to a day of the week. To be honest, I'm not sure why I was adamant about writing this way, but I was. I had only read a few blog posts before and certainly didn't follow anyone. Let's just say, I didn't know what I was doing.

Mommy Monday focused on all things mommy. The topics usually were along the lines of taking care of yourself, recipes, organization ideas, celebrations we were having or had and everyday family life.
Terrific Tuesday was the day I wrote about anything great in our lives.
Wellness Wednesday, I intended to focus on a Metabolism Miracle but found myself posting about other types of wellness as well. (Mental, spiritual, financial and physical are examples.)
Thoughtful Thursday focused on the current book I was reading or any "deep" thoughts I was having.

I did not blog Friday, Saturday or Sunday. Those were family days.

As time went on, Wellness Wednesday spread to other days, people turned to me for help from around the world, a Facebook page was created and ultimately a blog that solely focused on Wellness Wednesday. I named the blog NOW365. Needs or Wants 365. What does your body need today and what does your body want today? 365 days a year.

From the blog posts this book was born.

What is Metabolism B?

Diane Kress, the author of Metabolism Miracle is a registered award winning dietician. She believes that the main reason why all people do not lose weight the same way is because they all have different metabolisms. Her experiences have shown that about 50 percent of the people who come to counseling have metabolism B, also known as metabolic syndrome or insulin resistance which means an increased tendency of body to convert nutrients into body fat where a person with a normal metabolism would adsorb the nutrients or convert them into energy.

Steadyhealth.com explains that "resistance to insulin is usually the cause of type 2 diabetes, also called geriatric diabetes, but this resistance also occurs with type 1 diabetes, which is a major cause of heart diseases. Cells of patients who have resistance to insulin, no longer respond to the hormone insulin, which in normal conditions regulate glucose level in blood. Instead, glucose congests in the blood resulting in the fibrous plaque in coronary arteries. These deposits are the main cause of a range of cardiac diseases such as the heart attack. Among young women/girls insulin resistance allegedly causes polycystic ovary syndrome."

The symptoms of metabolism B are fatigue, lack of energy, fat on the abdomen and uncontrollable weight gain despite exercising. However there are many more than can make a woman feel she in menopausal, or cause one to be misdiagnosed with other disorders.

What I found interesting in my research was this analogy.

The main culprit for this is a process of carbohydrates degradation in the digestive system and insulin that regulates blood sugar.

This means that person with normal metabolism will feel full after eating a sandwich and have increased energy while the person suffering from metabolism B will crave something sweet a short time after eating because of sugar drop.

Why was this interesting to me?

Well, I look at the dessert menu at a restaurant before the main menu and always plan meals around desserts. If I don't have dessert at the end of a meal I might as well not have eaten.

Often, before reading that interesting fact, and while on numerous other diets I would work dessert into my allowed points for the day or calories. I know some of you can relate.

Metabolism B is more than those few symptoms listed above.

How about this checklist below located on the Metabolism Miracle website?

_____ You tire easily and frequently feel fatigued, even upon awaking.

_____ You feel mildly depressed.

_____ You feel an energy slump in the late afternoon.

_____ You frequently feel anxious.

_____ You crave carbohydrate foods, such as bread, chips, sweets, or pasta.

_____ Your midsection has a roll of fat., love handles, muffin top, or back fat

_____ You gain weight easily and find it difficult to lose weight.

_____ You have racing thoughts.

_____ Your sexual drive has declined or vanished

_____ You find it difficult to focus and concentrate and are easily distracted.

_____ You are irritable and have a "short fuse".

_____ You feel slightly dizzy, flushed, or "weak in the knees" after even a little bit of alcohol.

If you can check off any of these I plead with you to go to metabolismmiracle.com and take the full quiz.

The easiest way to sum up Metabolism B is to stress that a Met B body does not digest carbohydrates or convert insulin like a body with a normal metabolism.

The bad news is we have to eat differently than what we are used to. The good news is we should have been eating this way all along and now know what our bodies need.

Oxygen Mask

My very first blog post was written for moms. It used the analogy of flying with your child. The plane hits turbulence and the oxygen masks fall down in front of you. A mommy's instinct is to place the mask on their kids first, then their self. That is exactly what we are not supposed to do. Flight attendants explain in their per-flight instructions to place the mask on yourself first, then your child. We have to take care of ourselves before we can take care of anyone else.

How many of you do that? I don't.

The ultimate hypocrite. I can talk the talk but not walk the walk.

I'm learning and everyday is a struggle. One thing I will not do is give up.

I have seen first hand the effects of not taking care of yourself. They can be debilitating.

One of my best friends worked a stressful career in a hospital as a manager in Quality Control. Mayo clinic trained, she was an excellent floor nurse, surgical nurse, head nurse and ER nurse. She was off the floor and in an office. Making sure patients were cared for at the highest rate of care possible. Checking records of care, setting standards of care and educating those that performed the duties.

Late nights, weekends, early morning, skipped meals, and the overall stress of the job did her in when her body was attacked by an infection. This infection was so strong it attacked her heart. She ate gluten free, before gluten free was cool. She ate healthier than anyone I knew and still have ever known. She didn't smoke or drink. She exercised.

She was working at a new hospital when she got sick. Quality control was not great and the medical staff made many mistakes throughout her treatment. So many mistakes that she had to be flown by helicopter from Abilene, TX to Houston, TX. I am so proud of her for overcoming, for fighting. She could have died several times along the way.

The infection didn't care and when the "bad soldiers" took control of her body they did not surrender to the "good ones". They attacked and attacked. Eight years later she is on disability, her gait is still off and she has to work every day to keep what goals she has achieved.

I tell you this for many reasons. One is because before she moved to Abilene she was my neighbor. I was a young mom. She would work long, stressful hours and come home almost every day and walk straight to my house to get my kids so I could have relief. She was my first knowledge of having an oxygen mask. I was a better mom for her.

When she moved away I was solely dependent upon myself for relief and because of that I didn't make it a priority.

She also taught me by her illness that our bodies,too, need oxygen masks. Our bodies have a way of crying out for help. Most of us do not speak our bodies language, unfortunately. Most of the time when a body cries for an oxygen mask, for help, it cries so hard we, and even doctors, cannot decipher what it is trying to say.

You know what I mean. You've heard someone cry so hard that you cannot understand them. Bodies cry that hard, too.

When my dad was 40, he was at the highest point in his career. Recently promoted to Assistant Chief Patrol Agent of the United States Border Patrol in the Laredo, Texas, the largest inland port in the United States.

After a decade of being undercover, heading the ASU (Anti-Smuggling Unit), kicking in doors, running sting operations, getting death threats (to the point armed guards were placed at his front door and followed my step-mom everywhere she went) and bringing down entire smuggling rings he was now in the front office.

He knew he earned his place in his cushiony chair and window view of the main boulevard in Laredo.

One day they were holding a blood drive at his office. My dad gave blood with the rest, drank his juice and ate his cookies.

He went back to his office and began to feel bad so he went to the bathroom. He passed out. His body was crying for an oxygen mask but no one understood what it was saying.

Luckily, nurses were on site. He was stabilized there and rushed to the hospital where he was told nothing was wrong.

Over the course of a year he would have a series of these "episodes". They were strokes! The doctors referred to them, I think as "mini-strokes".

All the years of undercover work we would joke with him that he ate like a stoned teenager because when he would get home from a detail.

A detail was when he would follow a load of illegal aliens or drugs to a drop house and watch that house for a few days, building his case against the bad guys.

When he arrived home, as he got out of the car he had to kick through the ding-dong and honey bun wrappers, doughnut bags and coke cans to get his legs out of his undercover car, usually a Camaro or something cool like that.

He didn't eat this way anymore, he wasn't stressed like in his undercover days anymore but his body didn't know that. In fact, his body was just now able to cry out for help. It had spent so many years just trying to survive that when it was able to relax it didn't know what to do. (These are my opinions, definitely not medical opinions.)

He made changes to his diet and exercise regimen. He has now had 2 heart attacks. One he drove himself over 60 miles to the hospital.

His doctors still do not know exactly what is causing the heart attacks and do not know what caused the strokes. His body is crying but no one can understand what it is trying to say. If we knew where he needed his oxygen mask we would make those changes.

One final story, the hardest to tell, is the story of my husbands diagnosis of Trigeminal Neuralgia.

The Monday after Easter in 2010, we watched and felt a bump develop on the back of his head.

Soon, my husband was in so much pain that I had to take him to the emergency room. He was given a shot of Dilaudid and immediately went into cardiac failure.

He had an allergic reaction and his heart stopped.

By the grace of God he is here today. He has written a book about his triumphant journey overcoming Trigeminal Neuralgia, "Jesus Held Me".

His body was crying for and it literally took divine intervention to save him.

I thank God everyday for saving him and for holding him during that time.

A person with Metabolism B can and usually is misdiagnosed for many years.

Their bodies are desperately crying for help and no one can understand the cry.

Maybe you are going through menopause? Maybe you are depressed? Maybe you eat more than you think?

Metabolism B is referred to as The Great Masquerader for a reason.

Metabolism B sufferers rejoice because your oxygen mask in detailed in Metabolism Miracle.

I will share some details in the next chapter.

The Plan

The blogs have allowed me to reach out and help people that I would have never known. I've always heard the saying,"If I just help one person, it will be worth it." It is so true.

Receiving comments, emails, and texts from others thanking me for inspiring them or asking for advice is very rewarding. Once they see results, is the cherry on top.

However, writing the blog has presented me with an internal struggle.

How much of Dianne Kress' genius do I disclose? What can I legally disclose? Obviously, she wrote the book for income. I know she wrote Metabolism Miracle to help others, as well.

So, I turned to her internet site to see what she freely offered the public. I turned to other blogs to see what they had divulged. (Frankly, some said too much!)

It would be easy for me to type out the the "rules", allowed foods, etc. I could share all of the books recipes too. That would be cheating both sides. You and the author. If you suffer from Metabolism B (Hashimoto's thyroiditis, hypothyroid, insulin resistance, metabolic resistance, diabetes) you NEED more info than I can provide here.

What I really want to do is offer support to those following the plan and help those that are not yet following the plan get on board.

I am currently helping quite a few others on their journey and take their success very personal! Now I realize why personal trainers do what they do. Watching each transformation is amazing!

I'm proud of each and every one!

There are 3 steps with The Metabolism Miracle. I should be in step 3. Following this plan for about 4 months I have 30 inches off my body and about 20 pounds. I have cheated profusely! In fact, as of recently I have cheated so badly I think I want to start over with step 1 again. Truth be told— I never left step 1, it's very comfortable there. Oh, and I cheated so often that I had to keep adding 3 days to it and lost count.

STEP 1

8 weeks--A low-carb period to rest your overworked pancreas and liver while shrinking fat cells. Your energy will soar and you'll feel content. You will lose weight and your belly fat will slim down. The hard part? Not weighing daily. I'm definitely not defined by that number but it sure does motivate me. I'm not one to be disappointed by not seeing a loss or even a gain. If I've done what I'm supposed to do I know it will pay off in the end. For some, maybe you, not weighing yourself will be liberating. Relish in that. Enjoy it!

STEP 2

8 weeks or longer until you reach your desired weight~ Reintroduce healthy carbohydrates in the proper amount and at the right time, to promote continued fat burning and weight loss. Gently restart your rested pancreas and liver.
I can't say much more because I haven't done it yet!!!

STEP 3

Lifetime weight maintenance-- Opening your diet to more carbohydrates, including the treats that you may have been missing on Steps 1 & 2. Keeping your health and energy levels in tip-top shape and maintaining your weight loss permanently.

Other things:

EXERCISE: Intense exercise isn't necessary! 30 minutes of increased activity (it can be broken up throughout the day), 5 days a week. In the beginning I did a squat challenge, burpies, jumping jacks and crunches.

SLIP UPS: For a specific party or special occasion (a one time thing), don't change anything during the day to compensate for the party. Enjoy the party, eat what you want and then return to your plan by eating an appropriate snack before bedtime that very night! (no more than 1 slip up a week)

For a long weekend, holiday, or vacation~ eat what you want and then as soon as you get home, go through a quick 10 day detox (Step 1), followed by 10 days of reprogramming (Step 2).

HEALTHY FOODS: I don't have to buy any expensive diet shakes or weight-loss products. It is a rounded diet full of healthy veggies, protein, good fats, good carbs, etc.

VERY IMPORTANT:
WATER WATER WATER! Water flushes out the fat, literally!

A poem a wrote about the fat:

This little piggy went to market
This little piggy followed her diet
This little piggy had salad, nuts and cheese
This little piggy lost 1.5 pounds in a day
This little piggy's fat went wee wee wee out of her body!!!!!!

My favorite things to eat on Step 1:

nuts
cheese
meats
salads
low carb bread and tortillas

You can also have diet sodas, coffee, liquor and wine! I bought The Metabolism Miracle Cookbook that has tons of recipes. I NEED MY SWEETS and I always make sure to have plenty of the peanut butter cookies on hand, sugar free jello and whipped cream.

By following the steps in this book, I have seen remarkable improvements in my physical health. (20 pounds gone and 30 inches)

The book says mental and emotional health will improve as well. I'm still trying to get my thyroid function under control and know that has played a role in me not feeling 100% myself YET! But it's coming. I KNOW it is.

I hope this has helped you! I hope this gives a clearer picture of the diet plan. I look forward to answering any questions. Offering any assistance that I can!

My Story

Weight-loss by the month

Jan 2012------ 196

March   198

April   189

July   208

October   186

November	*180*
December	*176*
Jan 2013	*171*
February	*165*
March	*164 (started MM)*
April	*157*
May	*149*
June	*145*
August	*138*

Jaunuary(2014)-148

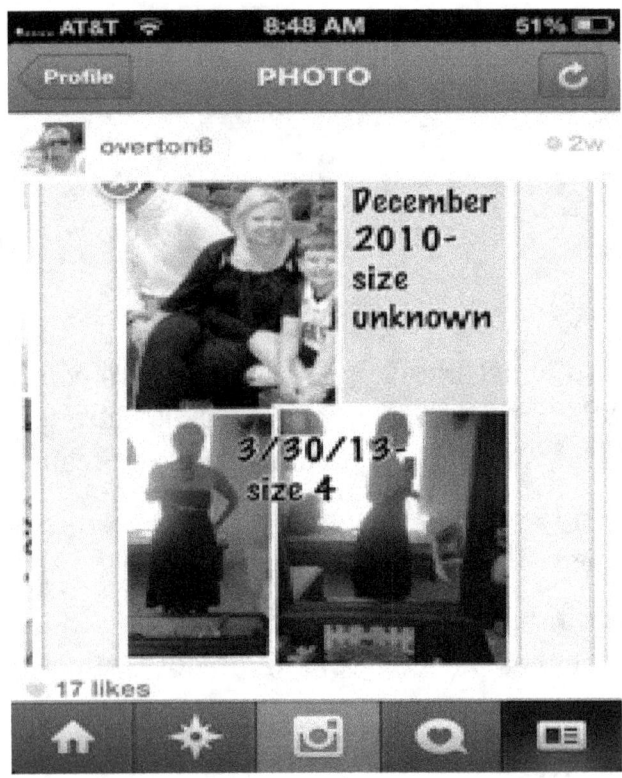

Several times in my 25 year struggle with thyroid problems I have been under-medicated, and over-medicated, and misdiagnosed.

My family history and that voice inside me are what kept me fighting to learn more about thyroid disease, as well as treatments for it. Hypothyroidism has effected both sides of my moms family and goes back generations.

My mom has Graves disease that went undiagnosed by "the best" endocrinologist in our area. It took her eyes literally bulging out of her head to get a diagnosis. My first diagnosis took me 2 years to get.

To those close to me, except my mom, I might have looked like I was a hypochondriac, going from doctor to doctor until they told me what I wanted to hear.

I did go from doctor to doctor until they told me what I wanted to hear but only because I knew something was wrong and I was going undiagnosed and I was not going to suffer like my mom and her sister. I wanted to learn, be proactive not reactive.

I have a very strong intuition. My father tells me I should have been an investigator. I often see things from angles that seemingly are crazy but turn out to be spot on.

For seven months of my second pregnancy my OB-GYN was insistent that my unborn child was a girl.

I told him every visit for 3 months that if the child is a girl something is wrong. I knew the child was not a girl.

All of my blood work was normal. There were no signs of any type of genetic disease, deformities,etc. But I KNEW, something was not right.

At seven months pregnant without any complications I had not decorated the nursery because of this reason. I knew my baby was healthy but was it twins? (I was huge!!) or a boy? So I begged to be placed in the sono-room at 30 weeks pregnant. As soon as the doppler touched my belly you could see my baby was a boy! I was not crazy!

When I was finally diagnosed with Hashimoto's Thyroiditis, my step-mother was with me. No one ever came with me to the doctor, in retrospect I think she came with me to make sure I wasn't crazy. As I said I was dead set on getting a diagnosis.

I had to travel over 200 miles to find a doctor who would take the time to listen to me. Every other doctor told me I was too young for thyroid issues at 22-24 years old, even though I exhibited almost every hypo symptom.

The day I was diagnosed with Hashimoto's thyroiditis was a relief! I was not crazy! I knew the journey ahead of me. Watching my mom and her sister suffer was not fun but I felt I could "cut it off at the pass", so to speak.

Well, I have managed to avoid Graves disease, yay!

However, the diagnosis of metabolic resistance, insulin resistance, pre-diabetes, fibromyalgia, etc. was not a diagnosis I ever thought I would get.

Believe me, when my doctor diagnosed all of those and a few more things on the same day in July of 2011, I kept her in the room for a while.

What medications did I have to take? Could I use herbs and oils instead? I wanted to know if I could have prevented these things. I wanted to know how to get rid of them. I wanted to find out what needed to be done to prevent my children from developing these issues.

If I'm being honest and I am, most of the the time to a fault, part of me took those diagnosis as an excuse to be fat. Heck, how could I lose weight with all of that going against me?

Soon, reality set in and I realized I didn't WANT to be fat and unhealthy, excuse or not. I work best turning a negative into a positive.

I was on a quest to defeat the fat.

The fat was winning!

Over a year after my diagnosis, injecting myself with expensive Byetta shots and eating healthy I was not any better off. I was the same weight, if not heavier.

I didn't know I was about to turn a big negative into a positive.

In 2012, I was struggling mentally and physically. I was fighting the biggest battle of my life, I had brain fog without the luxury of having it. I couldn't lose weight when my self image counted the most, my thyroid was out of whack, and I weighed a whopping 210-215 at 5'4".

My endo tried everything. I did what they said.

I tried countless diets for no less than 3- 6 months at a time The weight crept off.

Unfortunately, I was forced to visit a GP in my small town when my usual doctor turned their office into a membership only clinic and the membership cost $3000 a year plus office visits, etc.

I needed to prescription refills and my local GP was the easiest for that. I hoped he would follow my precious doctor's plan and I went prepared with all of my labs and notes from office visits.

I didn't get what I had hoped for in the office that day but in the end I got the answer I was looking for all along.

About 9 years earlier I weighed 180. The weight would not budge. I had 2 beautiful kids and was focused on mommy hood.

My brother 12 years younger with about 4 of his friends (I look at as either my own children or siblings) decided to wrestle me and give me a wedgie as they had years before. My brother went to grab my panties and came out with maw-maw underwear.

My brother threw me away saying, "Gross." The other boys left the room in hysterics or saying gross, making barf noises, etc. I was humiliated, angry (at myself) and surprisingly began to lose weight.

Going from 180 to 118 over the next few months with ease.

That was when I realized I'm motivated by humiliation as well as anger.

I would like to think I turn negatives into positives.

Back in the doctors office in our small town. This kid, maybe 30, proceeds to tell me, losing weight is simple. CALORIES IN= CALORIES OUT.

I politely said " I do not agree I have insulin resistance, metabolic syndrome , hypothyroid, Hashimoto's thyroiditis, have dieted for months without success, I am burning over 1000 calories a day exercising and have a massive amount of stress."

His response was this.--I do not write this to offend. I write this for numerous reasons. Please accept my apology in advance. Please know I have kept this as my secret because it is so disgusting and shameful.

Please know I cried at his words and merely walked out of his office because there was no sense in arguing with someone of that mentality. But also know within a few weeks I found Metabolism Miracle as a blessing from above. This story is why Metabolism Miracle is my passion.

No more hesitation…….

His words were this. "Cyndi, all that you have is on paper. But the truth remains the same. Too many doctors today give in to their patients, give them excuses to be fat, blame it on everything, make up medical terms to make excuses. But look at Nazi concentration camps. You didn't see fat people there. They were starved. Simple math. CALORIES IN= CALORIES OUT"

Those words still make me sick and cry.

Why would I repeat such disgusting thoughts? I want each of you that read this to know there is ignorance alive and well and it effects us. Unfortunately we cannot solely rely on our medical community to know what is right for us any more. The internet can do harm. It can create hypochondriacs. But it can save lives as it saved my husbands life (another story) and plenty more every day.

If I had not been so angry that day or humiliated I might not have looked so intently at the Thyroid Sexy Facebook page. I would not have found Metabolism Miracle.

His words pushed me to not give up.

DO NOT GIVE UP

DO NOT STAY WITH A DOCTOR THAT IS NOT HELPING YOU!

YOU DESERVE BETTER!

Hashimoto's thyroiditis, hypothyroid, insulin resistance, metabolic resistance, pre-diabetic (I guess goes with previous 2), 75 pounds over weight a doctor that basically told me to starve myself. I was frustrated and wanted to give up. The pounds had not budged. I had tried one diet after another in a 5 year period. I had never attempted low carb because years prior I did Atkins and gained weight!(after reading MM, I now know why)

I had tried:

Weight Watchers for the longest amount of time. The 4 hour body, The Lean, The 17 day diet, Perfect Weight America, Sugar Busters, You on a Diet, The Perricone Promise, whooo……those are the ones I remember.

Finally I began my own combination of diets and saw success. No guidelines. I just did what I thought worked for my body. Losing about 2-3 pounds a month was ok. Better than none and certainly better than gaining.

I knew there was something better.

One day in late February of 2013, while waiting for my kids to get out of school, I waited in the car as my baby slept in his car seat and I began reading Facebook. It wasn't anything out of the norm. I did this most days. I answered emails, phone calls and then played around on Facebook.

This day, God had a different plan. I like to think he was rewarding me for not losing it on the doctor and for not giving up for so long. I had kept my faith I would lose the weight to be healthy for my family.

Sometimes I was stronger than others. I always knew I would find an answer. I knew there was a way

There was! In a blurp, in a post on the Facebook page, Thyroid Sexy, I saw 2 words. Now it seems there was a golden glow around them. The words were "metabolism miracle".

Yes. I needed that. What was that, actually? Where do I find a metabolism miracle?

Metabolism had become a word I used daily.

"My metabolism is slow."

"I wish my metabolism worked."

Miracle was also a word I used daily.

I prayed for miracles in my life in various areas.

These two simple words combined together seemed—well, like a miracle.

I needed more information.

I did what I always do, an internet search. Oh gosh, just what I suspected. It was yet another diet. That's no miracle!!!!

My kids got into the car. I asked them about their day and our ride home commenced with Sophie and I singing our favorite song at the top of our lungs.

But the words kept going through my head…Metabolism miracle………metabolism miracle. A little bit later. Metabolism miracle.

So I went to my diet info place- sparkpeople.com. During the search I found some basic info. Nothing negative. My research continued for a few days.

Finally I bought the book and started reading it. I eventually decided it was a MIRACLE! The physics made sense, but and I mean BUT!!!!! It was low carb. Keep reading, I kept telling myself. I did.

Temporary low carb, then reintroduce carbs. Ok! I can do this.

Next obstacle? Convincing my husband I want to do yet another diet. I told him I needed to talk to him about a diet. He looked at me. I asked him to listen. I gave a concise as possible overview.

He said, "go for it with all my support".

YO YO MA NO MO

I just love that.

I do not yo-yo anymore.

Diane Kress stresses there is not a specific weight you must be. When you can easily maintain your weight, when your horrible symptoms go away and your blood work is normal you are at your ideal weight.

For me, it is not the 125 pounds I wanted.

This is my lifestyle now.

I have learned to gauge how I feel, by how I feel not by the numbers on the scale.

 In fact, I have not been on the scale in I while.

So my Metabolism Miracle journey began March 4, 2013.

Success was quick and easy. Dare I admit that?

Admitting success and not finding flaws in myself is not easy for me.

I could tell you my daily menu's.

I could also type out my daily weight (although we are not supposed to weigh daily).

I would only be doing those things to add fluff to this book.

I will tell you the fat melted off of me and it melted off quickly.

Your journey will be different than mine.

What you crave and enjoy will be different than what I craved and enjoyed.

I will add recipes at the end and offer help to anyone through my blogs, facebook and email at the end of the book.

What is important to me is that I stress how much Metabolism Miracle changes you from the the inside-out and the outside-in.

What it does for you will be different than what it has done for me.

For example, I have learned that eating peanuts in the morning is the best fuel for my system. I have learned that a huge salad at night is the perfect dinner.

Drinking water all day might keep me busy going to the potty but it really does melt the fat way.

As I pointed out 125 pounds is not where I ended up but my body truly found it's ideal weight naturally.

I eat what I want without feeling deprived or starving.

Mentally and physically I feel better.

You will too!

I would like to share a few successes:

I've often seen "before and after" pictures on Facebook and other forums that were amazing.

The visible differences really stood out.

I didn't think I was looking at me! The lady that took my picture asked me what I was doing differently.

I was able to tell her about Metabolism Miracle!

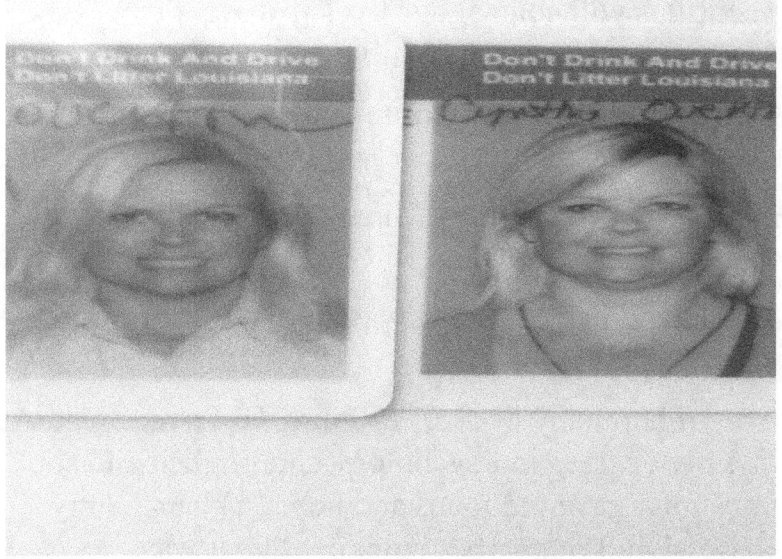

Another fun success was going bra shopping. Something I once disliked immensely turned into a lot of fun. Maybe it was going by myself? A very cold December day while in San Antonio, my husband sent me to Victoria Secret all alone to buy my first new bra in 2 years.

 I was excited! The store wasn't even opened yet when I arrived.

Taking my weekly measurements I had an idea of what size I needed so I grabbed a few when I walked in the door.

A saleslady rescued me! When all was said and done I wore a 32 DDD or a 34 DD.

One of my issues with losing almost 80 pounds was losing my breasts. I didn't want to. Apparently they just sag ALOT! They seemed so small, I guess they were compared to what they were before but walking out of there in a bra that supported the girls was honestly a great boost for me.

I tell you this story because it will be important for you along your journey to get fit and buy bras that lift and make you feel good about yourself. Before Metabolism Miracle or before the weight loss having a "good" support bra was not important to me. I didn't realize the difference in how I feel about myself. To be clear, I am not trying to be some VS model with boobs to my chin. My bra's had huge gaps in them where my breasts used to be. They would cave in from the empty space. What I mean by feeling good about myself is that I can feel comfortable in my clothes because my bra fits. It will be important, believe me.

Get Over Yourself

Insecurities used to eat me alive. Insecurities will control our lives if we let them and they had controlled mine for many years. To an extent they still do.

Then one day I read a few quotes written by one of my favorite authors of all time, Marianne Williamson, I felt a swift kick in the gut.

God showed me this quote in his time. Before Metabolism Miracle I would have shrunk into a deeper hole of insecurity.

Now, because of the great success of Metabolism Miracle I was able to read the quote and "digest" it from a different mindset.

I've often read her quotes and only one of her many books, A Return To Love. I read A Return To Love when I was 21 getting my degrees in Psychology and English and soul searching. A Return To Love saved my soul, gave me focus and hope, it changed my being. I hold that book as a prized possession. I remember buying it like it was yesterday.

When I was 21, I had not developed the insecurities that controlled me for so long. Holding the book as a prized possession did nothing for me. I should have been reading it all of these years.

It's like having a Bible next to your bed and never reading it. You aren't going to get anything out of it. We need to read the books than we feel a soul connection to throughout our life because at different stages in our lives our interpretations will be different.

The first quote I read is below:

"Our deepest fear is not that we are inadequate. Our deepest fear is that we are powerful beyond measure. It is our light, not our darkness that most frightens us. We ask ourselves, Who am I to be brilliant, gorgeous, talented, fabulous? Actually, who are you not to be? You are a child of God. Your playing small does not serve the world. There is nothing enlightened about shrinking so that other people won't feel insecure around you. We are all meant to shine, as children do. We were born to make manifest the glory of God that is within us. It's not just in some of us; it's in everyone. And as we let our own light shine, we unconsciously give other people permission to do the same. As we are liberated from our own fear, our presence automatically liberates others."

I've always seen her words as uplifting, guiding and comforting. Full of peace. Full of love.

Then I read the following quote:

"The solution to low self-esteem is to get over yourself and get a higher purpose."
~Marianne Williamson

First, I was angry.

Second, I prayed.

Third, I prayed, again.

Fourth, I did some soul searching.

So in essence low self esteem is actually the opposite? I don't have a higher purpose because I have low self esteem? I needed help so I typed in the quote as an Internet search. Not surprisingly this quote has a lot of negative comments attached to it in various locations. The more I read, the more I understood. Maybe she means something along the lines of this—When we dwell on our own shortcomings it gets us nowhere — when we find a higher cause or purpose, or feel useful in the world, it pulls us out of our problems, gives us a different outlook.

If you see if from the standpoint of the grass is always greener…..

Or if you have curly hair you want straight.

You have thin legs – you want muscular and vice versa.

Worrying about things you cannot control get's you no where.

Here's a quick random fact. Up until this summer I had not worn shorts out of the house in 8 years. In recent years I hadn't worn them at all. This summer I had to consciously decide to wear shorts and not wear sweats or jeans every day.

Some days I've cried leaving the house with shorts on because I'm so insecure about my legs. I tell myself "you weigh 137, wear a size 4-6 or small– get over it! Wear the shorts!" They are bermuda shorts, at that.

As stated above, it has been hard. Handsome hubby says, "you know you look good, you must, because you are wearing shorts."

I tried to explain to him the internal struggle I deal with. But unless you deal with the same type of insecurity you can't understand.

There are dimples. There is jiggling. I'm sure there is cellulite in the back where I can't see. All I can do is diet and exercise. If I don't then I'm to blame. If I do then I know I'm working on it.

 No, this is not an every day occurrence but if the occasion arises and shorts are more appropriate than jeans or sweats, I DO WEAR THEM!

I wish each and every one of you the same power. The power to tell yourself through the deep insecurities that you are beautiful, you are a God Spark.

All that is negative in your mind is not of love.

All that is not of love is not real, it is ego driven.

When we set our ego aside we leave room for the divine to step in.

When we stop focusing on our negatives, we leave room for positive.

You hear it everyday. A couple was trying to get pregnant and gave up. They adopted and she was pregnant within a few months.

When you aren't looking for a boyfriend or husband, you find the perfect person.

Well, when you let go of insecurities, they let go of you.

You will find positives you never knew existed. You will realize people are not even paying attention to you.

Reading my favorite author say to "get over myself" was a slap in the face. She was right! Truth be told, I am talking to me as much as I am talking to you right now, if not more.

We have to get over ourselves.

If you pick one thing to decide not to be insecure about anymore and truly make the decision not to be, I promise you, your life will change.

I do not make promises I cannot keep.

Ask my kiddos.....Remember every feeling we have is a choice.

Why would we WANT to feel bad.

I tell my kids, when we put ourselves down, we are telling God he did not create us "good enough". He created us in his image, perfectly imperfect humans.

Do you deal with insecurities?

How do you deal with them?

Do you feel you should get over yourself and find a higher purpose?

I believe we all need to seek a higher purpose whether we have low self esteem or not. Our reason for being is —-well—- our reason for being.

Man in the Mirror

If you don't like your current situation, your environment, your community, your world–look in the mirror.

I wrote this post about Michael Jackson on his birthday this year. It was important enough to me to add to this book.

Michael Jackson changed the world. Through his music, dancing, and philanthropy he was able to connect with every age group. Listen to his music. I bet you can remember specific moments in your life related to quite a few of his songs/ albums.

For Thoughtful Thursday I wanted to focus on "Man in the Mirror" it has taken me significantly longer to finish my post.

On a personal level, people often look at their life as insignificant, less than inspirational, going no where and maybe chose to complain instead of "making a change". Some of us continue to live as we were raised and some of us break the mold, break the cycle so to speak.

On a larger scale, we see horrific news items and turn the other cheek. We KNOW the state our family, our city, our state, our country, our world. But what can one person do?

We think we are only 1 and we are right. We are one GOD SPARK. One human being created to do extraordinary things.

God did not create us or we did not chose to be created to change every part of every bad situation at every level in our world. If we look at the big picture, the whole picture, it quite overwhelming. But if we break things down into tiny pieces they don't seem so daunting.

Yesterday I was helping my step daughter with her algebra homework. $4x-8=2x$ kinda thing. Each equation got more difficult. The process stayed the same but with more steps they became confusing and for her too much to handle. She said "I'll just save it for later." I replied, "No, let's gets this done." and showed her how to break the equations down to be as simple as the first. She got it!

If we have a desire to change something in the world break it down into a small piece. Accomplish that and continue to grow as you can.

Maybe you need to start with you. I know I "look in the mirror" everyday. In fact, as I've lost my patience as I've tried to write this post I've "looked in the mirror". Do I want to be an impatient mom for a blog? What's more important? Isn't social media an issue with families these days I try to keep away from? Boy, I probably "look in the mirror" way too much!

What would you change? How could you accomplish this?

I think Michael Jackson too "looked in the mirror". I think he tried to change the world, as well as be a great human being. Sometimes possibly way too critical of himself. I can't pretend to know.

His last years of his life were less than "normal". Some have said he gave so much love and all he ever wanted was to feel that love returned. Scandals enveloped his life. No need to rehash all of them. Child molestation questions scare me the most. Being abused as a child I pray that these allegations were false. If not, I pray for the children and for Michael. But he has met his maker and dealt with whatever needed to be dealt with. The research I did for this post said that "Man in the Mirror" was one of Micheal's favorites. I hope Michael liked what he saw when he looked in the mirror. Sadly, I think not. For that I pray he has found peace.

For you, the reader of this book, I pray you find what you are looking for. I pray you do not suffer any longer from your ailments and the Metabolism Miracle as well as My Metabolic Miracle help you along your journey.

Amen

Tips and Tricks

There are several important tips. These tips will save you time, money, energy, frustration, and ultimately your life. No, I am not being dramatic. The effects of Metabolism B can kill you. We must do our part by taking responsibility for our body and do something. In some cases, if you do not follow these "tips" you will not be following the plan. I decided to add them as tips because some of us are still hard headed. I am one of them and catch myself slipping back into my old habits. I say this often, when I write, I am talking to myself as much as the reader. A few examples for me are not eating often enough and not drinking enough water. I will focus mostly on tips for step 1 for purposes of this book. There are different tips for each step.

1. DO NOT WAIT TO START. Do not wait for the holidays to be over. Do not wait until Monday. Do not wait for your birthday or vacation to go by. Start NOW. The beauty of MM is it forgives! If you cheat, just add 3 days.

2. Drink water! If you drink the required water (64 ounces) you will see inches disappear before your eyes. The pounds do not matter as much as the inches!

3. To eat every 5 hours for me means that I need to plan my meals for every 3-4 because things happen. If you think you are leaving the house and will be back in time to eat I recommend packing a snack. Never leave home without nuts and water!

4. Eat protein at every meal. Eat as much as you can. Eat it until you cannot eat any more!

5. Take a good multivitamin.

6. Get "natural" vitamins when possible. People with metabolic issues often have difficulty absorbing vitamin d. I was prescribed 10,000 iu a day for a month then I took it 3 times a week. A body cannot adsorb that much, even pharmaceutical grade. (my opinion) Get out in the sun! Do you know that the occurrences of skin cancer have risen since the usage of sun screen has risen. (That is another book)

7. Do not eat nuts from the tall plastic canister. They have an additive that needs to be counted in the 5x5. The small tins are best if you do not want to shell your nuts.

8. For a great snack buy nuts you need to shell. They take longer to eat and you do not risk having additives.

9. Sign up to Metabolism Miracles website. Pay the membership fee if you can. She is updating the book and posts those updates to her subscribers.

10. Do not discount the effects of physical exercise. Do not worry about cardio. Weight bearing- squats, pushups, etc are what you want to worry about. Keeping your muscle mass is important. Use your muscles to keep your muscles.

11. Exercise first thing in the morning, 25 jumping jacks, 25 squats, 25 crunches and stretches. It will take 5 minutes and will boost your metabolism tremendously for the rest of the day.

12. Relax every day. Meditate if possible.

13. Think positive and reflect on your accomplishment. Try on clothes you haven't been able to wear in a long time. You will be surprised how quickly the fat melts off.

14. Get your family on board with you. I did it without mine knowing. I made Metabolism Miracle dinners without letting them know that is what it was. It was so much easier on me.

15. LOW CARB BREAD and TORTILLA's buy them and keep them on hand at all times!

16. If you wake up in the night, EAT!

17. If you cannot eat as I cannot squirt whipped cream in your mouth with a spoonful of sugar-free. Anything. Like that will do. Please try this. It really helps your metabolism.

18. Traveling is completely doable. You have to plan, be prepared and want to do it. My sister-in-law lost more weight/inches when she traveled then when she was at home because she could control what food she was around easier.

19. Find a cheerleader and use them.

20. More importantly be a cheerleader!

21. Take progress photos. I failed at this because I was so embarrassed. I wish I would have taken them now.

22. Reread the book over and over. You think you know it. You think you understand but there are small tid-bits of info that you will overlook. For me it was having to have fiber in 5x5 for step one.

23. Upon doctors approval, of course, drink caffeine! Yes, green tea or coffee even diet soda but not too many.

24. For every beverage you consume that is not water add that many more ounces of water to your daily allotment.

25. Add flaxseed oil to your meals, salads, etc. to burn more of the yucky brown fat.

26. Do not eat Cool-Whip. You must count the carbs in it. Eat the Reddi-whip Whipped cream or make your own with fresh whipping cream and splenda, whip it up until it forms peaks.

27. Use butter, all the butter you want.

28. If you don't have doctor restrictions don't worry about lean meats. I ate bacon and sausage and lost tons of fat. In fact, it seemed the more fat I ate the more I lost.

29. DO NOT GIVE UP! Look for positive changes. Look for progress. You will see them!

30. Onions, garlic, bells peppers and cheese do wonders to a meat that has become boring.

31. Flaxseed oil and coconut oil are wonderful to cook with and have metabolism boosting properties.

32. Eat what you want when you want it. If you crave meat in the morning, eat it. If you want eggs at night, eat them at night. Your body will be going through many changes and you will crave things that you will be very surprised about. Go with it. This is one of the reason I find it difficult to give a meal plan or ideas because I have found that each person I have helped craves different things. One person who never liked salmon all of a sudden began craving it. Someone else I've helped rejoiced in the glory that she could enjoy her favorite chicken salad again after years of avoiding it because of the mayo content.

Water, agua, wasser, eau, vann, voda

No matter how you say water. Water is one of the best things we can put in our bodies on a daily basis. Here are a few reasons why……

Drinking water helps you lose weight because it flushes down the by-products of fat breakdown.

Drinking water reduces hunger, it's an effective appetite suppressant so you'll eat less. Plus, water has zero calories.

Natural Remedy for Headache: Helps to relieve headache and back pains due to dehydration. Although there are many other reasons that contribute to headache, dehydration is the common one.

Look Younger with Healthier Skin: You'll look younger when your skin is properly hydrated. Water helps to replenish skin tissues, moisturizes skin and increases skin elasticity.

Better Productivity at Work: Your brain is mostly made up of water, thus drinking water helps you think better, be more alert and concentrate more.

Better Exercise: Drinking water regulates your body temperature. You'll feel more energetic when doing exercises and water helps to fuel your muscles.

Helps in Digestion and Constipation: Drinking water raises your metabolism because it helps in digestion. Fiber and water go hand in hand so that you can have your daily bowel movement.

Less Cramps and Sprains: Proper hydration helps keep your joints and muscles lubricated, so you'll less likely get cramps and sprains.

Less Likely to Get Sick and Feel Healthy: Drinking plenty of water helps fight against flu and other ailments like kidney stones, heart attack, arthritis, etc. Water added with lemon is used for ailments like respiratory disease, intestinal problems, rheumatism and arthritis etc. In other words, one of the benefits of drinking water can improve our immune system.

Relieves Fatigue: Water is used by the body to help flush out toxins and waste products from the body. If your body lacks water, your heart, for instance, needs to work harder to pump out the oxygenated blood to all cells. The rest of the vital organs have to work harder as well. Your organs will be exhausted and so will you.

Good Mood: Your body feels good and you will too.

Reduce the Risk of Cancer: Some studies show that drinking a healthy amount of water may reduce the risks of bladder cancer and colon cancer. Water dilutes the concentration of cancer-causing agents in the urine and shortens the time in which they are in contact with bladder lining.

**DRINK COLD WATER German researchers found that drinking 6 cups of cold water a day (that's 48 ounces) can raise resting metabolism by about 50 calories daily—enough to shed 5 pounds in a year. The increase may come from the work it takes to heat the water to body temperature. Though the extra calories you burn drinking a single glass doesn't amount to much, making it a habit can add up to pounds lost with essentially zero additional effort.

Will you drink more now?
How much do you currently drink? Personally I do not drink nearly enough. Some days none at all, if we are being honest.

A few recipes

Life Saving Peanut Butter Cookies
Ingredients
1 cup sucralose, plus more for dipping the fork
1 large egg

1 teaspoon vanilla extract
1 cup creamy or chunky NATURAL peanut butter
1 teaspoon baking soda

Instructions:
1. Preheat the oven to 350 degrees. Spray pan with cooking spray.
2. Mix the sweetener, egg and vanilla with an electric mixer on low for 3 minutes in a medium bowl. Add the peanut butter and baking soda. Mix on medium speed until the dough comes together, about 30 seconds.
3. Form the dough into walnut size balls and place them 2 inches apart on the baking sheet.
4. Dip the fork in the artificial sweetener and flatten the cookies with crisscross marks
5. Bake for 10-12 minutes, until lightly browned.

Cool.

Eat these alone or with whipped cream. You can even spray the whipped cream on one, place another on top, place in the freezer and its like an ice cream sandwich.

Another version is to cream 4 ounces of cream cheese with 4 ounces of natural peanut butter. Use that to put on top or to make them into sandwiches.

Other recipe ideas:
Jalapeno Poppers- I called them Bear Claws 20 years ago
Half a fresh jalapeno, scrape out the veins and seeds, use gloves, no water while scraping them out.
Once cleaned wash them.
Add a generous amount of cream cheese seasoned with seasonal all, tony chacheres, or another type of seasoning you like
Place a fresh peeled shrimp on top of the cream cheese.
Wrap with ½ slice of thin bacon
Bake in the oven at 350 degrees until done or BBQ.

Wrap chicken with bacon and marinade in Newman's Own Olive Oil and Vinaigrette salad dressing. Bake in the oven or grill
Wrap sliced beef around a slivered jalapeno, marinade in Newman's Own Olive Oil and Vinaigrette salad dressing and grill.

Green Bean Bundles:
Fresh green beans
cream cheese

jarred sliced jalapenos
bacon
Take 3 green beans, place a teaspoon or so of cream cheese on top, place a jalapeno slice on top, wrap with bacon and grill or bake. Season with your favorite all purpose seasoning.

Tortilla ideas:
Keep it flat and place all of the regular pizza fixings you would use except for pizza sauce.

Melt mexican cheese and chicken in a tortilla folded in half (quesadilla)
To kick it up a notch saute it in a little seasoned butter (Land o Lakes Saute Express)

Spinach Madeline
Servings
4-6

Ingredients
2 (10 ounce) boxes frozen spinach, cooked and drained
(reserve 1/2 cup liquid)
2 tablespoons flour
onion, chopped(medium size)
1 (6 ounce)
garlic cheese rolls, cut into small pieces (this is cheese NOT BREAD)
1/4 cup butter
salt & pepper
1/2 cup evaporated milk
3/4 teaspoon garlic salt
1 tablespoon Worcestershire sauce
1 dash hot sauce (Louisiana Fish Fry brand or favorite)
Directions:

1 Melt butter, add onions and flour; stir until smooth.
2 Add the milk and mix well.
3 Add the rest of the seasonings and 1/2 of the cheese roll, and stir until cheese melts.
4 Combine all ingredients in casserole.
5 Bake at 350 for 20-25 minutes
6 Serve along side chicken , salmon, pork chops, anything!

Nut butters:
2 cups of your favorite nuts, toasted
2 tbsp of olive oil or flaxseed oil

salt to taste

Mix in a food processor until blended to the texture you want. Add more or less oil depending upon your taste.

Cauliflower Poppers:

Cut and clean cauliflower

drizzle the florets with olive oil and sprinkle with salt and pepper.

Bake at 350 until brown and caramelized, about 30 minutes.

These are great for snacking.

In closing, I would like to thank you for buying this book. I would like to offer my assistance if you at all need or want it. I would love your reviews and feedback.

You can contact me through:

Facebook at Metabolism Miracle Living, Cyndi Overton

Instagram at overton6,

Twitter @cyndioverton

Now365.wordpress.com

simplycynful.wordpress.com